ENDOMETRIOSIS PLANT BASED DIET COOKBOOK

OVER 20 RECIPES TO REDUCE INFLAMMATION NATURALLY, RELIEVE SYMPTOMS AND RESTORE PRODUCTIVE LIFE

KAREN EDMONDS

TABLE OF CONTENT

STAY
HOPEFUL

INTRODUCTION

The idea for this "Endometriosis Plant-Based Diet Cookbook" may be found in the quiet corners of resilience, where health and flavour intersect. This culinary adventure is more than simply a collection of recipes; it's a story woven with strands of empowerment, healing, and the transformational power of plant-based nourishment.

Consider Karen, a woman navigating the complex maze of endometriosis, dealing with pain, tiredness, and the search for a long-term solution. Karen began on a personal quest after becoming dissatisfied with traditional therapies and empowered by the growing amount of information demonstrating the influence of nutrition on endometriosis symptoms. This cookbook arose from her kitchen, demonstrating the significant link between plant-based nutrition and endometriosis management.

Karen found a variety of nutrients capable of not only tantalising taste sensations but also supporting hormonal balance and lowering inflammation as she toured bright farmers' markets and experimented with nature's bounty. Each dish is a chapter in her story: a triumph over adversity, a celebration of adopting a plant-based diet, and a call to those on a similar path.

This cookbook is a caring guide in addition to its tantalising fragrances and wonderful flavours. It digs into the science of endometriosis, investigates the symbiotic link between plant-based diet and hormonal balance, and provides a road map for individuals looking for peace in the embrace of nutritious, nourishing meals. Let us embark on a culinary adventure that goes beyond just nourishment, creating a story of wellness, resilience, and the transforming potential of plant-based life.

CHAPTER 1:
UNDERSTANDING ENDOMETRIOSIS

Endometriosis is a complicated and sometimes misunderstood ailment that affects millions of women worldwide. This section seeks to shed light on its complexities, including the description, causes, symptoms, and diagnosis, as well as the critical role diet plays in managing this difficult illness.

Definition and Causes:

Endometriosis is a persistent medical disorder in which endometrium, or tissue akin to the uterine lining, develops outside the uterine cavity. This misaligned tissue reacts to hormonal fluctuations, causing inflammation, discomfort, and adhesion development. Endometriosis's exact cause is unknown, however ideas include retrograde menstruation, immune system malfunction, and genetic predispositions. Determining the reasons is essential for developing successful management methods.

Diagnosis and Symptoms:

Endometriosis causes a variety of symptoms, including pelvic discomfort and menstrual abnormalities, as well as gastrointestinal and urine difficulties. Unfortunately, the variety of symptoms frequently results in misdiagnosis or delayed detection. Clinical assessment, imaging investigations, and occasionally laparoscopic surgery for visual confirmation are used to make a diagnosis. Early identification is critical for prompt care and better quality of life for people who are impacted.

The Importance of Nutrition in Endometriosis Management:

Nutrition is emerging as a critical component in the overall care of endometriosis. Certain foods have anti-inflammatory characteristics and can help to regulate hormones, potentially relieving symptoms. A plant-based diet high in antioxidants, omega-3 fatty acids, and fibre may help to reduce inflammation and provide comfort. Understanding nutrition's enormous influence encourages individuals to take an active role in their well-being, supplementing standard medical measures.

When navigating the maze of endometriosis, information serves as a compass. Individuals may engage on a path towards educated decision-making and a more empowered, resilient journey through the challenges of endometriosis by understanding the nature of the condition, its origins, symptoms, and the effect of nutrition.

STAY
HOPEFUL

CHAPTER 2: THE BENEFITS OF PLANT-BASED CHOICE

Adopting a plant-based diet has special benefits for people traversing the difficult terrain of endometriosis. While everyone's experience with endometriosis is different, adopting a plant-centric diet can provide significant advantages that help with symptom management and general well-being. Here are some significant ways that plant-based nutrition coincides with the requirements of persons suffering with endometriosis:

Anti-Inflammatory support:

Anti-inflammatory chemicals are naturally abundant in plant-based diets. Endometriosis is characterised by chronic inflammation, which contributes to pain and discomfort. Individuals may notice a drop in inflammatory indicators by emphasising

13

fruits, vegetables, nuts, seeds, and whole grains, thus easing symptoms.

Hormonal Balance:

Hormonal changes, notably oestrogen, impact endometriosis. Plant-based diets include phytoestrogens, (found in flaxseeds, soy, lentils, and whole grains) which are plant chemicals that have estrogen-like properties. These chemicals may aid in the modulation of hormonal activity, resulting in a more balanced hormonal environment.

Fibre for Digestive Health:

A fiber-rich diet, high in plant-based foods, promotes digestive health. Fibre promotes regular bowel motions and can help control endometriosis-related gastrointestinal symptoms such as bloating and constipation.

Nutrient Density and Overall Health:

Plant-based diets provide a wide range of vital elements, such as vitamins, minerals, and antioxidants. These nutrients contribute to general well-being by strengthening the immune system, energy levels, and resilience—all of which are important for those dealing with endometriosis.

Reduced Hormone and Additive Exposure:

Plant-based diets often include less animal products, which may have additional hormones and other chemicals. Individuals with endometriosis may be able to better control their hormonal balance if they limit their exposure to these chemicals.

Weight Management and discomfort Reduction:

In endometriosis patients, maintaining a healthy weight is connected with less inflammation and discomfort. Plant-based diets, which are frequently lower in calorie density and saturated fats, can help with weight control and may help with discomfort sensations.

Increased Omega-3 Fatty Acids:

Plant-based omega-3 fatty acid sources such as flaxseeds, chia seeds, and walnuts can help maintain a healthy omega-3 to omega-6 fatty acid ratio. This balance is related with anti-inflammatory effects, which may provide comfort to patients suffering from endometriosis.

Holistic Wellness and Emotional Resilience:

Plant-based nutrition promotes mental and emotional well-being as well as physical health. Plant-derived nutrients can improve mood and emotional resilience, which are crucial parts of managing the emotional toll of chronic illnesses like endometriosis.

While there is little or no treatment for endometriosis, a plant-based diet provides a complete and holistic strategy for treating symptoms and boosting overall well-being. Plant-based diet becomes a great ally in the road to relief and resilience when used as part of a holistic strategy.

CHAPTER 3: BREAKFASTS FOR BALANCED HORMONES

Energizing Smoothie Bowls

Berry Bliss Bowl

Ingredients:

- 1 cup of mixed berries (strawberries, blueberries, raspberries)
- 1 ripe banana
- 1/2 cup of almond milk
- 1 tablespoon of chia seeds
- 1 tablespoon of almond butter
- Toppings: granola and fresh berries

Instructions:

- Blend mixed berries, banana, almond milk, chia seeds, and almond butter until smooth.
- Put into a bowl and top with granola and fresh berries. This bowl is high in

antioxidants, fibre, and healthy fats, making it a tasty and nutritious way to start the day.

Nutritional values (approx. per serving):

Calories: 250-300

Protein: 5-8 grams

Fat: 10-15 grams

Carbohydrates: 35-40 grams

Fiber: 8-10 grams

Sugars: 15-20 grams (mostly from natural fruit sugars)

Vitamin C: 50-70% of daily recommended intake

Antioxidants: High levels from berries and chia seeds

Calcium: 10-15% of daily recommended intake

Iron: 5-8% of daily recommended intake

Green Goddess Power Smoothie

Ingredients:

- 1 cup of spinach leaves
- ½ cucumber, peeled and sliced
- ½ avocado
- ½ cup of pineapple chunks
- 1 tablespoon of fresh mint leaves
- 1 cup coconut water
- Optional: Chia seeds for garnish

Instructions:

- Mix spinach, cucumber, avocado, pineapple, mint, and coconut water in a blender. Blend until creamy.
- Transfer into a bowl, garnish with chia seeds if preferred, enjoy the energising combination of greens and tropical sweetness. This smoothie bowl is a delightful way to start your morning, packed with vitamins, minerals, and hydrating coconut water.

Customisation Suggestions:

- For an extra protein boost, add a scoop of plant-based protein powder.
- Try alternative toppings, such as chopped almonds, hemp seeds, or shredded coconut.
- Adjust the thickness of the smoothie to your liking by altering the amount of liquid (almond milk, coconut water).
- For an extra nutritious boost, add hormone-balancing nutrients like maca powder or flaxseed.

Nutritional values (approx. per serving):

Calories: 200-250

Protein: 4-6 grams

Fat: 12-15 grams

Carbohydrates: 25-30 grams

Fiber: 7-9 grams

Sugars: 15-18 grams (mostly from natural fruit sugars)

Vitamin A: 30-40% of daily recommended intake

Vitamin C: 60-80% of daily recommended intake

Potassium: 20-25% of daily recommended intake

Magnesium: 15-20% of daily recommended intake

Nutrient-Packed Overnight Oats

Chocolate Almond Butter Overnight Oats

Ingredients:

- 1/2 cup old-fashioned oats
- 1/2 cup unsweetened almond milk (or plant-based of choice)
- 1 tablespoon cocoa powder, unsweetened
- 1 tablespoon of almond butter

- 1 tablespoon maple syrup or sweetener of choice
- 1/2 teaspoon of vanilla extract
- A pinch of salt
- Sliced bananas and a sprinkle of chopped almonds for topping

Instructions:

- Combine oats, almond milk, chocolate powder, almond butter, maple syrup, vanilla extract, and a bit of salt in a jar or airtight container.
- Stir thoroughly to ensure that all ingredients are evenly distributed.
- Refrigerate the jar or container overnight or for at least 4 hours.
- To get a creamy consistency, give the mixture a vigorous swirl before serving.
- To add texture and flavour, top with sliced bananas and a sprinkling of chopped almonds.

Nutritional Values (approx. per serving):

Calories: 400-450

Protein: 10-15 grams

Fat: 20-25 grams

Carbohydrates: 45-50 grams

Fiber: 8-10 grams

Sugars: 12-15 grams

Calcium: 15-20% of daily recommended intake

Iron: 10-15% of daily recommended intake

Tropical Chia Seed Pudding

Ingredients:

- 1/4 cup chia seeds
- 1 cup coconut milk (or plant-based milk of choice)
- 1 tablespoon maple syrup or sweetener of choice
- 1/2 teaspoon of vanilla extract
- 1/2 cup of pineapple, chopped
- 1/2 cup of mango, diced
- 1 kiwi, peeled and sliced

- Shredded coconut and a few mint leaves for garnish

Instructions:

- In a mixing dish, combine the chia seeds, coconut milk, maple syrup, and vanilla extract.
- Allow the mixture to settle for 5 minutes before whisking again to prevent clumping.
- Refrigerate the dish for at least 2 hours or overnight to allow the chia seeds to absorb the liquid and form a pudding-like consistency.
- Stir before serving to achieve an equal texture.
- Chia seed pudding should be layered with diced pineapple, mango and sliced kiwi.
- Garnish with shredded coconut and mint leaves if preferred

Nutritional Values (approx. per serving):

Calories: 350-400

Protein: 7-10 grams

Fat: 20-25 grams

Carbohydrates: 40-45 grams

Fiber: 12-15 grams

Sugars: 20-25 grams

Vitamin C: 80-100% of daily recommended intake

Calcium: 20-25% of daily recommended intake

Iron: 10-15% of daily recommended intake

Hearty Breakfast Quinoa Bowls

Southwest Quinoa Breakfast Bowl

Ingredients:

- 1/2 cup of cooked quinoa
- 1/4 cup of black beans, washed and drained

- 1/4 cup corn kernels (fresh, frozen, or canned)
- 1/2 sliced avocado
- 1/4 cup cherry tomatoes, halved
- 1 tablespoon fresh cilantro, chopped
- 1 tablespoon lime juice
- Salt and pepper to taste
- Hot sauce or salsa for extra flavour (optional)

Instructions:

- Combine cooked quinoa, black beans, corn, avocado slices and cherry tomatoes in a mixing dish.
- Drizzle the lime juice over the ingredients and toss to incorporate gently.
- Season to taste with salt and pepper.
- Garnish with fresh cilantro and, if preferred, a dab of spicy sauce or salsa.

Nutritional Values (approx. per serving):

Calories: 350-400

Protein: 10-15 grams

Fat: 15-20 grams

Carbohydrates: 45-50 grams

Fiber: 10-12 grams

Sugars: 3-5 grams

Vitamin C: 15-20% of daily recommended intake

Calcium: 5-8% of daily recommended intake

Iron: 10-15% of daily recommended intake

Mediterranean Chickpea Quinoa Bowl

Ingredients:

- 1/2 cup cooked quinoa
- 1/2 cup canned chickpeas, washed and drained
- 1/4 cup cucumber, diced
- 1/4 cup cherry tomatoes, halved
- 1/4 cup of sliced Kalamata olives, sliced

- 2 tablespoons finely cut red onion
- 2 tablespoons feta cheese, crumbled (optional)
- Fresh parsley, chopped, for garnish
- Extra virgin olive oil for drizzling
- Lemon wedges for serving

Instructions:

- Combine cooked quinoa, chickpeas, cucumber, cherry tomatoes, olives, and red onion in a mixing bowl.
- To combine the ingredients, gently toss them together.
- Sprinkle feta cheese on top if using.
- Drizzle with extra virgin olive oil.
- Garnish with fresh parsley if desired.
- Serve with lemon wedges on the side for an added citrus flavour boost.

Nutritional Values (approx. per serving):

Calories: 350-400

Protein: 12-15 grams

Fat: 15-18 grams

Carbohydrates: 40-45 grams

Fiber: 8-10 grams

Sugars: 3-5 grams

Vitamin C: 20-25% of daily recommended intake

Calcium: 6-8% of daily recommended intake

Iron: 10-15% of daily recommended intake

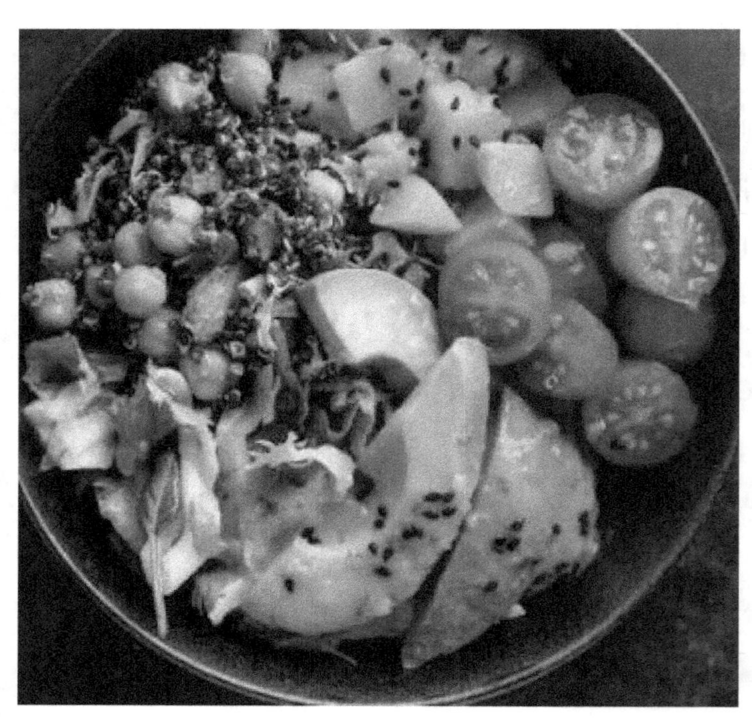

CHAPTER 4: NOURISHING LUNCHES FOR ENDOMETRIOSIS RELIEF

Salads with Hormone-Balancing Ingredients

Kale and Pomegranate Salad with Citrus Dressing

Ingredients:

For the Salad:

- 4 cups of fresh kale, stems removed and leaves cut
- 1 cup of pomegranate seeds
- 1/4 cup chopped walnuts
- 1/4 cup crumbled feta cheese (optional)
- 1/4 cup of thinly sliced red onion

For the Citrus Dressing:

- 3 tablespoons of extra virgin olive oil

- 1 tablespoon of fresh orange juice
- 1 tablespoon of fresh lemon juice
- 1 teaspoon of honey or maple syrup
- Salt and pepper to taste

Instructions:

Prepare the Salad:

- Combine the chopped kale, pomegranate seeds, walnuts, feta cheese (if using), and sliced red onion in a large mixing basin.
- Gently toss the ingredients to combine evenly.

Make the Citrus Dressing:

- Whisk together the extra virgin olive oil, fresh orange juice, fresh lemon juice, honey or maple syrup, salt, and pepper in a small bowl.
- Adjust the seasoning to suit your taste.

Assemble the Salad:

- Drizzle the salad with the citrus dressing.

- Toss the salad with the dressing until the items are evenly covered.

Serve:

- Divide the salad among serving basins or plates.
- Garnish with more pomegranate seeds and feta cheese, if preferred.

Nutritional Values (approx. per serving):

Calories: 300-350

Protein: 7-10 grams

Fat: 20-25 grams

Carbohydrates: 30-35 grams

Fiber: 8-10 grams

Sugars: 15-20 grams

Vitamin C: 120-150% of daily recommended intake

Calcium: 10-15% of daily recommended intake

Iron: 8-10% of daily recommended intake

Roasted Vegetable Quinoa Salad

Ingredients:

For the Salad:

- 1 cup of quinoa, cooked and cooled
- 2 cups of mixed vegetables (e.g., bell peppers, zucchini, cherry tomatoes, red onion), sliced
- 2 tablespoons of olive oil
- 1 teaspoon of dried herbs (such as oregano, thyme, or rosemary)
- Salt and pepper to taste
- 1/4 cup crumbled feta cheese (optional)
- Fresh parsley or basil, chopped, for garnish

For the Lemon-Herb Dressing:

- 3 tablespoons of extra virgin olive oil
- 2 tablespoons of fresh lemon juice
- 1 teaspoon Dijon mustard
- 1 clove of minced garlic
- Salt and pepper to taste

Instructions:

Prepare the roasted vegetables as follows:

- Preheat the oven to 400 degrees Fahrenheit (200 degrees Celsius).
- Toss the chopped vegetables with the olive oil, dry herbs, salt, and pepper in a large mixing dish.
- Place the vegetables on a baking sheet in an equal layer and roast for 20-25 minutes, or until soft and gently browned. To ensure even roasting, stir halfway through.

Cook the Quinoa as follows:

- Cook the quinoa according to package directions in a separate pot. Allow to cool to room temperature after cooking.

To prepare the Lemon-Herb Dressing:

- Whisk together the extra virgin olive oil, fresh lemon juice, Dijon mustard, minced garlic, salt, and pepper in a small bowl. Place aside.

Prepare the Salad:

- Combine the cooked and cooled quinoa with the roasted vegetables in a large mixing bowl.
- Dress the quinoa and vegetables with the Lemon-Herb Dressing. Gently toss everything to coat evenly.

Serve:

- Serve the salad on a dish or individual plates.
- Optional: Sprinkle with crumbled feta cheese on top.
- Garnish with fresh parsley or basil if desired.

Nutritional Values (approx. per serving):

Calories: 400-450

Protein: 10-15 grams

Fat: 20-25 grams

Carbohydrates: 45-50 grams

Fiber: 7-9 grams

Sugars: 5-8 grams

Vitamin C: 60-80% of daily recommended intake

Calcium: 6-8% of daily recommended intake

Iron: 10-15% of daily recommended intake

Satisfying Plant-Based Protein Lunches

Lentil and Sweet Potato Stew

Ingredients:

- 1 cup dry green or brown lentils, washed and drained
- 2 medium sweet potatoes, peeled and diced
- 1 onion, chopped
- 2 carrots, diced
- 2 celery stalks, chopped
- 3 cloves of minced garlic
- 1 can (14 oz) diced tomatoes, undrained
- 4 cups of vegetable broth
- 1 teaspoon of ground cumin
- 1 teaspoon of ground coriander

- 1/2 teaspoon of smoked paprika
- 1/2 teaspoon of turmeric
- Salt and pepper to taste
- 2 tablespoons of olive oil

Fresh parsley or cilantro for garnish

Instructions:

Sauté the Aromatics:

- Warm the olive oil in a big saucepan over medium heat.
- Sauté the chopped onion and minced garlic until softened and aromatic.

Put Vegetables and Spices:

- Add the chopped sweet potatoes, carrots, and celery.
- Mix in the cumin, coriander, smoked paprika, turmeric, salt, and pepper. Mix well to coat the vegetables with the seasonings.

Cook Lentils:

- Place washed lentils in a saucepan and cover with vegetable broth.

- Bring the mixture to a boil, then lower to a low heat.
- Cover and cook for 20-25 minutes, or until the lentils are cooked.

Add Tomatoes:

- Add the undrained diced tomatoes to the saucepan and stir to incorporate.
- Continue to cook for another 10-15 minutes to enable the flavours to mingle.

Season to taste and serve:

- Season with salt and pepper to taste.
- Ladle the stew into serving dishes and top with fresh parsley or cilantro

Nutritional Values (per Serving):

Calories: 350-400

Protein: 15-18 grams

Fat: 6-8 grams

Carbohydrates: 60-65 grams

Fiber: 15-18 grams

Sugars: 10-12 grams

Vitamin A: 200-250% of daily recommended intake

Vitamin C: 20-25% of daily recommended intake

Iron: 15-20% of daily recommended intake

Chickpea and Spinach Curry

Ingredients:

- 1 can (15 oz) of chickpeas, washed and drained
- 2 cups of fresh spinach leaves, washed and cut
- 1 onion, chopped
- 2 tomatoes, finley chopped
- 3 cloves of minced garlic
- 1-inch ginger, grated
- 1 can (14 oz) coconut milk
- 2 tablespoons of curry powder
- 1 teaspoon of ground cumin
- 1 teaspoon of ground coriander

- 1/2 teaspoon turmeric
- 1/2 teaspoon red chili flakes (to taste)
- Salt and pepper to taste
- 2 tablespoons of cooking oil
- Fresh cilantro for garnish
- Cooked brown rice or quinoa for serving

Instructions:

Sauté Aromatics:

- Heat the cooking oil in a big pan over medium heat.
- Sauté the chopped onions until they are transparent.

Put Garlic and Ginger:

- Mix in the minced garlic and ginger. Cook for another minute, or until aromatic.

Add Spices:

- Combine curry powder, ground cumin, ground coriander, turmeric, red chilli flakes, salt, and pepper in a mixing bowl. Mix well to coat the onions with the seasonings.

Add Chickpeas and Tomatoes:

- Add the chickpeas and tomatoes to the pan. Cook for 5-7 minutes, or until the tomatoes begin to soften.

Add the Coconut Milk:

- Pour in the coconut milk and mix to blend all of the ingredients.
- Allow the curry to boil for 15-20 minutes to allow the flavours to combine and the sauce to thicken.

Spinach should be added:

- When the curry has thickened, stir in the spinach. Stir the spinach into the curry until it wilts and is equally distributed.

Season to taste and serve:

- Season the curry with salt and pepper to taste.

- Over cooked brown rice or quinoa, serve the Chickpea and Spinach Curry.
- Garnish with fresh cilantro if preferred.

Nutritional Values (approx. per serving):

Calories: 400-450

Protein: 10-12 grams

Fat: 20-25 grams

Carbohydrates: 45-50 grams

Fiber: 10-12 grams

Sugars: 5-8 grams

Vitamin A: 80-100% of daily recommended intake

Vitamin C: 30-40% of daily recommended intake

Iron: 15-20% of daily recommended intake

Turmeric Ginger Carrot Soup

Ingredients:

- 1 pound carrots, peeled and chopped
- 1 onion, finely chopped
- 3 cloves of minced garlic
- 1 tablespoon of grated fresh ginger
- 1 teaspoon of ground turmeric
- 1/2 teaspoon of ground cumin
- 1/4 teaspoon cayenne pepper (to taste)
- 4 cups of vegetable broth
- 1 can (14 oz) coconut milk
- 2 tablespoons of olive oil
- Salt and pepper to taste
- Fresh cilantro or parsley for garnish
- Toasted pumpkin seeds for topping (optional)

Instructions:

Sauté Aromatics:

- Warm the olive oil in a big saucepan over medium heat.

- Cook until the onions are transparent.

Add Garlic and Ginger:

- Mix in the minced garlic and ginger. Cook for another minute, or until aromatic

Add Spices:

- Mix in the turmeric, cumin, cayenne pepper, salt, and pepper. Mix well to coat the onions with the seasonings.

Cook Carrots:

- Stir in the chopped carrots to blend with the fragrant mixture.
- Cook for 5-7 minutes, or until the carrots soften.

Pour in Broth and Coconut Milk:

- Combine the vegetable broth and coconut milk in a mixing bowl. To blend, stir everything together.
- Bring the mixture to a boil, then lower to a low heat.

- Cook, covered, for 15-20 minutes, or until the carrots are soft.

Blend the Soup:

- Blend the soup with an immersion blender or in batches in a blender until smooth and creamy.

Season to taste and Serve:

- Season the soup with salt and pepper to taste.
- Pour into serving dishes and top with fresh cilantro or parsley.
- To add crunch, sprinkle with roasted pumpkin seeds.

Nutritional Values (approx. per serving):

Calories: 250-300

Protein: 3-5 grams

Fat: 20-25 grams

Carbohydrates: 15-20 grams

Fiber: 4-6 grams

Sugars: 5-8 grams

Vitamin A: 300-400% of daily recommended intake

Vitamin C: 15-20% of daily recommended intake

Iron: 8-10% of daily recommended intake

Creamy Broccoli and White Bean Soup

Ingredients:

- 2 cups of broccoli florets
- 1 can (15 oz) white beans, washed and drained
- 1 onion, finely cut
- 2 cloves of minced garlic
- 1 medium potato, peeled and diced
- 4 cups of vegetable broth
- 1 cup of unsweetened almond milk (or plant-based milk of choice)
- 2 tablespoons of olive oil

- 1 teaspoon of dried thyme
- Salt and pepper to taste
- Squeeze of lemon juice (optional)
- Fresh chives or parsley for garnish

Instructions:

Sauté Aromatics:

- Warm the olive oil in a big saucepan over medium heat.
- Cook until the onions are transparent.

Add Garlic and Potato

- Mix in the minced garlic and potato dices. Cook for another 2-3 minutes.

Add Broccoli and White Beans:

- Fill the saucepan with broccoli florets and white beans. Combine with the aromatics.

Pour in Broth and Almond Milk:

- Combine vegetable broth and almond milk in a mixing bowl. To blend, stir everything together.

- Bring the mixture to a boil, then lower to a low heat.
- Cook, covered, for 15-20 minutes, or until the vegetables are soft.

Blend the Soup:

- Blend the soup with an immersion blender or in batches in a blender until smooth and creamy.

Season and Finish:

- Season with salt and pepper to taste after adding the dry thyme.
- If preferred, add a squeeze of lemon juice to brighten the dish.

Serve:

- Pour the creamy soup into individual bowls.
- Garnish with fresh chives or parsley if desired.

Nutritional Values (approx. per serving):

Calories: 250-300

Protein: 8-10 grams

Fat: 10-12 grams

Carbohydrates: 35-40 grams

Fiber: 8-10 grams

Sugars: 3-5 grams

Vitamin A: 150-200% of daily recommended intake

Vitamin C: 100-120% of daily recommended intake

Iron: 10-15% of daily recommended intake

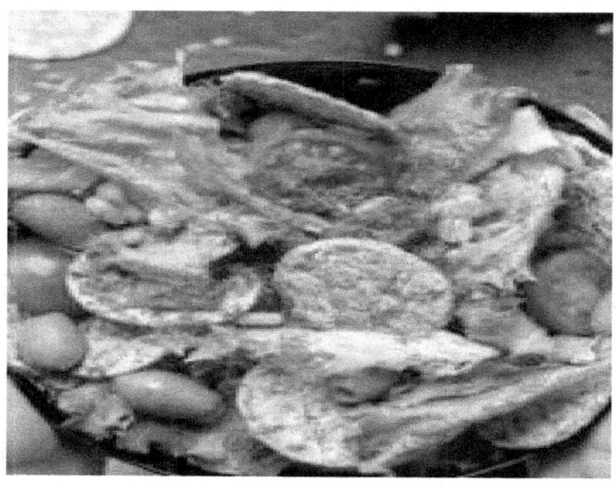

CHAPTER 5: ENDOMETRIOSIS-FRIENDLY DINNERS

Wholesome One-Pot Meals

Quinoa and Black Bean Skillet

Ingredients:

- 1 cup quinoa, washed
- 2 cups of vegetable broth
- 1 can (15 oz) black beans, washed and drained
- 1 bell pepper, diced (any color)
- 1 onion, finely chopped
- 2 cloves of minced garlic
- 1 cup of corn kernels (fresh, frozen, or canned)
- 1 teaspoon of ground cumin
- 1 teaspoon of chili powder
- 1/2 teaspoon smoked paprika
- Salt and pepper to taste
- 2 tablespoons of olive oil

- Fresh cilantro or green onions for garnish
- Avocado slices for topping (optional)
- Lime wedges for serving

Instructions:

Cook Quinoa:

- Warm the olive oil in a big pan over medium heat.
- Sauté the chopped onions until they are translucent

Add Garlic and Bell Pepper:

- Combine minced garlic and diced bell pepper in a mixing bowl. Cook for another 2-3 minutes, or until the peppers soften.

Add Quinoa and Black Beans:

- Stir rinsed quinoa into the aromatic mixture in the pan.
- Add black beans and veggie broth. Combine thoroughly.

Season and Cook:

- Sprinkle the quinoa mixture with cumin, chilli powder, smoked paprika, salt, and pepper. Stir to distribute the spices evenly.
- Cover the skillet and cook for 15-20 minutes, or until the quinoa is tender and the liquid has been absorbed.
- Stir in the corn kernels and let them to cook through for another 2-3 minutes.

Garnish and Serve:

- Garnish with fresh cilantro or green onions if desired.
- Top with avocado slices if desired.
- Serve with lime wedges on the side for a zesty blast of freshness.

Nutritional Values (approx. per serving):

Calories: 350-400

Protein: 10-12 grams

Fat: 10-12 grams

Carbohydrates: 55-60 grams

Fiber: 8-10 grams

Sugars: 4-6 grams

Vitamin C: 60-80% of daily recommended intake

Iron: 15-20% of daily recommended intake

Sweet Potato and Lentil Curry

Ingredients:

- 1 cup of dry green or brown lentils, washed and drained
- 2 big sweet potatoes, peeled and diced
- 1 onion, finely chopped
- 3 cloves of minced garlic
- 1-inch grated ginger
- 1 can (14 oz) of diced tomatoes, undrained
- 1 can (14 oz) of coconut milk
- 2 tablespoons of curry powder
- 1 teaspoon of ground cumin
- 1 teaspoon of ground coriander
- 1/2 teaspoon of turmeric
- 1/2 teaspoon of red chili flakes (to taste)

- Salt and pepper to taste
- 2 tablespoons of cooking oil
- Fresh cilantro for garnish
- Cooked brown rice for serving

Instructions:

Sauté Aromatics:

- Heat the cooking oil in a big pot over medium heat.
- Sauté the chopped onions until they are translucent.

Add Garlic and Ginger:

- Mix in the minced garlic and grated ginger. Cook for another minute, or until aromatic.

Add Spices:

- Add curry powder, ground cumin, ground coriander, turmeric, red chilli flakes, salt, and pepper to taste. Mix thoroughly to coat the onions with the spices.

Cook Lentils and Sweet Potatoes:

- Add rinsed lentils, diced sweet potatoes, In a large pot, combine rinsed lentils, diced sweet potatoes, diced tomatoes, and coconut milk. To combine, stir everything together.
- Bring the mixture to a boil, then reduce to a low heat.
- Cover and cook for 20-25 minutes, or until the lentils and sweet potatoes are tender.

Adjust Seasoning and Serve:

- Taste the curry and adjust the seasoning as needed.
- Serve the Sweet Potato and Lentil Curry over cooked brown rice or with naan.
- Garnish with fresh cilantro.

Nutritional Values (approx. per serving):

Calories: 400-450

Protein: 15-18 grams

Fat: 15-20 grams

Carbohydrates: 55-60 grams

Fiber: 12-15 grams

Sugars: 8-10 grams

Vitamin A: 400-500% of daily recommended intake

Vitamin C: 30-40% of daily recommended intake

Iron: 15-20% of daily recommended intake

Comforting Pasta Dishes

Zucchini Noodles with Tomato Basil Sauce

Ingredients:

For the Zucchini Noodles:

- 4 medium-sized zucchini, spiralized into noodles
- 2 tablespoons olive oil
- 2 cloves of minced garlic
- Salt and pepper to taste

For the Tomato Basil Sauce:

- 2 cups of cherry tomatoes, chopped
- 3 tablespoons of tomato paste
- 2 tablespoons of fresh basil, chopped
- 2 cloves of minced garlic
- 1 tablespoon of olive oil
- Salt and pepper to taste
- Red pepper flakes for a spicy kick(optional)
- Optional Toppings:
- Grated Parmesan cheese or nutritional yeast
- Pine nuts or chopped walnuts
- Fresh basil leaves for garnish

Instructions:

Prepare the Zucchini Noodles:

- Using a spiralizer, spiralize the zucchini into noodles.
- Warm the olive oil in a big saucepan over medium heat.
- Sauté the minced garlic for 1-2 minutes, or until aromatic.
- Toss the zucchini noodles with the garlic in the pan.

- Cook for 3-5 minutes, or until the noodles are soft. Season to taste with salt and pepper.
- Set aside after removing from the heat.

Make the Tomato Basil Sauce:

- In a separate pan, heat the olive oil over medium heat.
- Sauté the minced garlic for 1-2 minutes.
- Cook until the cherry tomatoes begin to soften.
- Add tomato paste, fresh basil, salt, and pepper to taste. Add red pepper flakes if you prefer it hot.
- Cook for another 5-7 minutes, or until the tomatoes have broken down and the sauce has thickened.

Combine Noodles and Sauce:

- Serve the zucchini noodles with the tomato basil sauce.
- Gently toss the noodles in the sauce to coat evenly.

Serve:

- Individually dish the Zucchini Noodles with Tomato Basil Sauce.
- Top with grated Parmesan cheese or nutritional yeast, pine nuts or chopped walnuts, and fresh basil leaves, if desired.

Nutritional Values (approx. per serving):

Calories: 150-200

Protein: 5-8 grams

Fat: 10-12 grams

Carbohydrates: 15-20 grams

Fiber: 5-8 grams

Sugars: 10-12 grams

Vitamin C: 40-50% of daily recommended intake

Vitamin A: 20-30% of daily recommended intake

Creamy Avocado and Spinach Pasta

Ingredients:

- 8 oz (227g) whole-grain or gluten-free pasta
- 2 ripe avocados, peeled and pitted
- 2 cups of fresh spinach leaves, washed
- 3 cloves of minced garlic
- 1/4 cup of fresh basil leaves, cut
- 1/4 cup fresh parsley, cut
- 1/4 cup of pine nuts, toasted
- 1/4 cup of nutritional yeast (optional)
- 1 lemon, juiced
- 3 tablespoons of extra virgin olive oil
- Salt and pepper to taste
- Red pepper flakes for a spicy kick (optional)
- Cherry tomatoes for garnish (optional)

Instructions:

Cook the Pasta:

- Cook the pasta according to the package directions until it is al dente.
- Before draining the pasta, save about 1/2 cup of the cooking water.

Prepare the Avocado Sauce:

- Combine the peeled and pitted avocados, fresh spinach, minced garlic, chopped basil, chopped parsley, toasted pine nuts, nutritional yeast (if using), lemon juice, and extra virgin olive oil in a blender or food processor.
- Blend until the mixture is smooth and creamy. If the sauce is too thick, thin it with some of the remaining pasta cooking water to achieve the correct consistency.
- Season the sauce to taste with salt and pepper. If desired, add red pepper flakes for a spicy kick.

Combine Pasta and Sauce:

- Coat the cooked pasta in the creamy avocado and spinach sauce.

Serve:

- Individually dish the Creamy Avocado and Spinach Pasta.
- If desired, garnish with halved cherry tomatoes.
- Drizzle with extra virgin olive oil and top with more pine nuts if desired.

Nutritional Values (approx. per serving):

Calories: 400-450

Protein: 10-12 grams

Fat: 20-25 grams

Carbohydrates: 50-60 grams

Fiber: 8-10 grams

Sugars: 3-5 grams

Vitamin C: 30-40% of daily recommended intake

Vitamin A: 20-30% of daily recommended intake

Balanced Grain Bowls

Teriyaki Tempeh Brown Rice Bowl

Ingredients:

For the Teriyaki Tempeh:

- 1 pack of (8 oz) tempeh, cut into cubes
- 1/4 cup of soy sauce or tamari (for a gluten-free option)
- 2 tablespoons of maple syrup or agave nectar
- 1 tablespoon vinegar (rice)
- 1 teaspoon of sesame oil
- 2 cloves of minced garlic
- 1 teaspoon of grated ginger
- 1 tablespoon of corn starch (optional, for added thickness)
- 2 tablespoons of cooking oil

For the Brown Rice Bowl:

- 1 cup of brown rice, cooked
- 1 cup of broccoli florets, steamed
- 1 carrot, shredded

- 1/2 red bell pepper, thinly cut
- 1/4 cup of edamame, shelled
- Sesame seeds for garnish
- Green onions, chopped, for garnish
- Crushed red pepper flakes for a spicy kick (optional)

Instructions:

Marinate and Cook the Tempeh:

- To make the teriyaki marinade, combine soy sauce, maple syrup, rice vinegar, sesame oil, chopped garlic, and grated ginger in a mixing bowl.
- Toss the tempeh cubes in the marinade to coat well. Allow at least 15-20 minutes for it to marinade.
- In a pan over medium heat, heat the cooking oil. Cook until the marinated tempeh cubes are golden brown on all sides. If you want a thicker sauce, combine cornflour and a little water in a small bowl and add it to the pan.

Assemble the Bowl:

- On top of the rice, layer steamed broccoli, shredded carrots, sliced red bell pepper, and edamame.

Top with Teriyaki Tempeh:

- Serve the teriyaki tempeh cubes over the prepared vegetables and rice.

Garnish and Serve:

- Sprinkle the dish with sesame seeds and chopped green onions.
- Crushed red pepper flakes can be used for a spicy kick if desired.
- Immediately serve the Teriyaki Tempeh Brown Rice Bowl.

Nutritional Values (approx. per serving):

Calories: 450-500

Protein: 20-25 grams

Fat: 15-18 grams

Carbohydrates: 60-70 grams

Fiber: 8-10 grams

Sugars: 8-10 grams

Vitamin C: 80-100% of daily recommended intake

Iron: 15-20% of daily recommended intake

Mexican-Inspired Cauliflower Rice Bowl

Ingredients:

For the Cauliflower Rice:

- 1 big riced cauliflower (or 4 cups pre-riced cauliflower)
- 1 tablespoon of olive oil
- 1 teaspoon of ground cumin
- 1 teaspoon of chili powder
- 1/2 teaspoon of paprika
- Salt and pepper to taste

For the Bowl:

- 1 can (15 oz) of black beans, washed and drained

- 1 cup of corn kernels (fresh, frozen, or canned)
- 1 cup of cherry tomatoes, halved
- 1 avocado, sliced
- 1/2 red finely sliced onion
- Fresh cilantro leaves for garnish
- Lime wedges for serving

For the Dressing:

- 2 tablespoons of olive oil
- 1 lime, juiced
- 1 teaspoon of ground cumin
- Salt and pepper to taste

Instructions:

Prepare the Cauliflower Rice:

- If you are not using pre-riced cauliflower, chop it into florets and pulse it in a food processor until it resembles rice.
- In a large pan over medium heat, heat the olive oil.

- Combine the riced cauliflower, ground cumin, chilli powder, paprika, salt, and pepper in a mixing bowl.
- Sauté the cauliflower for 5-7 minutes, or until it is cooked but not mushy. Place aside.

Assemble the Bowl:

- Serve the cauliflower rice in separate dishes.

Toppings are optional.

- On top of the cauliflower rice, layer black beans, corn kernels, cherry tomatoes, avocado slices and chopped red onion.

Prepare the Dressing:

- Whisk together the olive oil, lime juice, ground cumin, salt, and pepper in a small bowl.

Drizzle with Dressing:

- Dress the Mexican-Inspired Cauliflower Rice Bowl with the dressing.

Garnish and Serve:

- Garnish with fresh cilantro leaves and serve.
- Serve with lime wedges on the side for an additional zesty flavour boost.

Nutritional Values (approx. per serving):

Calories: 350-400

Protein: 10-12 grams

Fat: 20-25 grams

Carbohydrates: 40-45 grams

Fiber: 15-18 grams

Sugars: 8-10 grams

Vitamin C: 60-80% of daily recommended intake

Iron: 10-15% of daily recommended intake

CHAPTER 6: HORMONAL SNACKS AND SIDE DISHES

Energy-Boosting Snacks

Almond and Date Energy Bites

Ingredients:

- 1 cup of raw, unsalted almonds
- 1 cup of pitted Medjool dates
- 2 tablespoons of almond butter
- 1 tablespoon of chia seeds
- 1 tablespoon of flaxseeds (ground)
- 1/2 teaspoon vanilla extract
- A pinch of salt
- Shredded coconut or sesame seeds for coating (optional)

Instructions:

Prepare the Almonds:

- Pulse the almonds in a food processor until finely crushed, approximating coarse almond flour. Place aside.

Mix Ingredients:

- In a food processor, combine ground almonds, pitted Medjool dates, almond butter, chia seeds, ground flaxseeds, vanilla essence, and a sprinkle of salt.

Prepare the Mixture:

- Mix the ingredients together until they create a sticky, homogeneous dough. You should be able to simply squeeze the mixture together.

Form into Bites:

- Scoop tiny amounts of the mixture and roll it between your palms to make bite-sized balls.

Optional Coating:

- Roll the energy bites in shredded coconut or sesame seeds if preferred for an added layer of flavour and texture.

Set and chill:

- Refrigerate the energy bites for at least 30 minutes to allow them to firm up.

Keep and Enjoy:

- Transfer the Almond and Date Energy Bites to an airtight container after they have hardened.
- Keep refrigerated for up to two weeks.

Nutritional Values (approx. per serving - 2 bites):

Calories: 150-200

Protein: 4-6 grams

Fat: 9-12 grams

Carbohydrates: 18-22 grams

Fiber: 4-6 grams

Sugars: 12-15 grams

Calcium: 6-8% of daily recommended intake

Iron: 8-10% of daily recommended intake

Guacamole Ingredients:

- 3 ripe avocados
- 1 small finely diced red onion
- 1-2 tomatoes, diced
- 1 jalapeño, seeded and minced
- 2 cloves of minced garlic
- 1/4 cup fresh cilantro, chopped
- 2 limes, juiced
- Salt and pepper to taste
- *Vegetable Sticks*:
- Carrot sticks
- Cucumber spears
- Bell pepper strips (assorted colors)
- Celery sticks

Instructions:

Prepare the Guacamole:

- Cut the avocados in half, remove the pits, and scoop the flesh into a bowl.

- With a fork or potato masher, mash the avocados until smooth, leaving some pieces for texture.
- To the mashed avocados, add diced red onion, tomatoes, minced jalapeo, minced garlic, chopped cilantro, and lime juice.
- Combine everything until fully blended.
- Season to taste with salt and pepper. As required, adjust the lime juice or salt.

Prepare the Vegetable Sticks:

- Carrot sticks, cucumber spears, bell pepper strips, and celery sticks should be washed and sliced into sticks.

Serve:

- Place the Guacamole in a serving dish and serve.
- Arrange the different vegetable sticks around the dish for dipping.

Optional garnish:

- To add a bright touch, garnish the Guacamole with more cilantro or chopped tomatoes.

Snack Time:

- Enjoy this fresh and tasty snack by dipping the vegetable sticks into the guacamole.

Nutritional Values (approx. per serving):

Calories: 150-200

Protein: 3-5 grams

Fat: 12-15 grams

Carbohydrates: 10-15 grams

Fiber: 6-8 grams

Sugars: 2-4 grams

Vitamin C: 30-40% of daily recommended intake

Folate: 15-20% of daily recommended intake

Hormone balancing

Turmeric Roasted Cauliflower

Ingredients:

- 1 large head of cauliflower, cut into florets
- 2 tablespoons of olive oil
- 1 teaspoon of ground turmeric
- 1 teaspoon of ground cumin
- 1/2 teaspoon of ground coriander
- 1/2 teaspoon of paprika
- 1/2 teaspoon of garlic powder
- Salt and pepper to taste
- Fresh cilantro or parsley for garnish (optional)
- Lemon wedges for serving

Instructions:

Preheat the Oven:

- Preheat your oven to 425°F (220°C).

Cauliflower should be prepared as follows:

- Cut the cauliflower into bite-sized florets, making sure they are all around the same size for even roasting.

To make the Turmeric Spice Blend:

- Combine olive oil, ground turmeric, ground cumin, ground coriander, paprika, garlic powder, salt, and pepper in a small bowl. Mix well to make a vivid turmeric spice blend.

Coat the Cauliflower:

- Line a baking sheet with parchment paper or a silicone baking mat and place the cauliflower florets on top.
- Drizzle the turmeric spice mixture over the cauliflower florets and toss to coat evenly.

Bake in the Oven:

- Bake the cauliflower for 20-25 minutes, or until the edges are golden brown and the cauliflower is soft. To ensure consistent cooking, toss halfway during the roasting time.

Garnish and serve with:

- Turn off the oven and set aside the Turmeric Roasted Cauliflower.
- If preferred, garnish with fresh cilantro or parsley.
- For a zesty boost, serve with lemon slices on the side.

Nutritional Values (approx. per serving):

Calories: 100-150

Protein: 4-6 grams

Fat: 7-9 grams

Carbohydrates: 10-12 grams

Fiber: 4-6 grams

Sugars: 3-5 grams

Vitamin C: 80-100% of daily recommended intake

Vitamin K: 15-20% of daily recommended intake

Lemon Garlic Quinoa

Ingredients:

- 1 cup of washed quinoa
- 2 cups of vegetable broth or water
- Zest of 1 lemon
- 1-2 lemons, juiced (adjust to taste)
- 3 cloves of minced garlic
- 2 tablespoons of olive oil
- Salt and pepper to taste
- Fresh parsley for garnish (optional)

Instructions:

Rinse the Quinoa thoroughly:

- To eliminate any bitterness, rinse the quinoa under cold running water.

Cook the Quinoa as follows:

- Combine the washed quinoa and vegetable broth or water in a medium saucepan.
- Bring to a boil, then lower to a low heat, cover, and cook for 15-20 minutes, or

until the quinoa is tender and the liquid has been absorbed.

Make the Lemon Garlic Sauce:

- While the quinoa is cooking, mix together the olive oil, minced garlic, lemon zest, and lemon juice in a small bowl.

Toss the Quinoa:

- When the quinoa has finished cooking, fluff it with a fork to separate the grains.

Quinoa with Lemon Garlic Mixture:

- Pour over the cooked quinoa the lemon garlic mixture.

Toss and season:

- Season with salt and pepper to taste.
- Toss the quinoa with the lemon garlic mixture until thoroughly incorporated.

Garnish and serve:

- If preferred, garnish with fresh parsley.

- Serve as a savoury side dish with the Lemon Garlic Quinoa.

Nutritional Values (approx. per serving):

Calories: 200-250

Protein: 5-7 grams

Fat: 7-9 grams

Carbohydrates: 30-35 grams

Fiber: 3-5 grams

Sugars: 1-2 grams

Vitamin C: 20-30% of daily recommended intake

Iron: 10-15% of daily recommended intake

CHAPTER 7: DESSERTS OPTIONS

Chocolate Avocado Mousse

Ingredients:

- 2 ripe avocados, peeled and pitted
- 1/4 cup of cocoa powder (unsweetened)
- 1/4 cup maple syrup or agave nectar
- 1 teaspoon of vanilla extract
- A pinch of salt
- 1/4 cup of almond milk or any non-dairy milk
- Optional toppings: Fresh berries, chopped nuts, or a dollop of coconut whipped cream

Instructions:

Make the Avocados:

- Scoop the flesh from the ripe avocados into a blender or food processor.

Mix in the cocoa powder and sweetener:

- To the avocados, add cocoa powder, maple syrup or agave nectar, vanilla essence, and a sprinkle of salt.

Blend until completely smooth:

- Blend the ingredients together until they are smooth and creamy. As required, scrape down the sides of the blender or food processor.

Sweetness should be adjusted as follows:

- Adjust the sweetness of the mousse as needed by adding extra maple syrup or agave nectar.

Include Almond Milk:

- While the blender or food processor is working, slowly drizzle in the almond milk (or other nondairy milk of choice) until the mousse achieves the desired consistency. You may need to come to a halt and scrape down the sides once again.

Mousse should be chilled:

- Place the Chocolate Avocado Mousse in individual serving dishes or glasses.
- Refrigerate the mousse for at least 30 minutes to allow it to cold and firm.

Garnish and serve:

- Garnish with fresh berries, chopped nuts, or a dollop of coconut whipped cream before serving.

Nutritional Values (approx. per serving):

Calories: 200-250

Protein: 3-5 grams

Fat: 15-20 grams

Carbohydrates: 20-25 grams

Fiber: 7-10 grams

Sugars: 10-15 grams

Vitamin C: 10-15% of daily recommended intake

Iron: 10-15% of daily recommended intake

Berry and Coconut Bliss Balls

Ingredients:

- 1 cup of mixed berries (strawberries, blueberries, raspberries)
- 1 cup of pitted Medjool dates
- 1 cup of shredded coconut (unsweetened)
- 1/2 cup of rolled oats
- 1/4 cup of chia seeds
- 1 teaspoon of vanilla extract
- A pinch of salt
- Additional shredded coconut for coating (optional)

Instructions:

Make the Berries:

- If using fresh berries, properly wash them. If using frozen berries, allow to defrost before use.

Combine the following ingredients:

- Combine mixed berries, pitted Medjool dates, shredded coconut, rolled oats, chia seeds, vanilla essence, and a touch of salt in a food processor.

Mix until a dough forms:

- Mix the ingredients together until they create a sticky, homogeneous dough. The mixture should hold together when you pinch it.

Form into balls:

- Scoop out little amounts of the mixture and roll it between your palms to make bite-sized bliss balls.

Coating Options:

- Roll the bliss balls in extra shredded coconut if desired for a textured coating.

Set and chill:

- Refrigerate the Berry and Coconut Bliss Balls for at least 30 minutes to allow them to firm up.

Keep and Enjoy:

- Transfer the bliss balls to an airtight container after they have hardened.
- Keep refrigerated for up to two weeks.

Nutritional Values (approx. per serving - 2 bliss balls):

Calories: 150-200

Protein: 2-4 grams

Fat: 7-9 grams

Carbohydrates: 20-25 grams

Fiber: 4-6 grams

Sugars: 14-18 grams

Vitamin C: 10-15% of daily recommended intake

Iron: 6-8% of daily recommended intake

CHAPTER 8: ENDOMETRIOSIS LIFESTYLE MANAGING TIPS

Endometriosis management necessitates a multifaceted strategy that extends beyond medical therapy. Implementing lifestyle modifications can considerably help to alleviate symptoms and improve general well-being. Here are some lifestyle suggestions for dealing with endometriosis:

A well-balanced diet:

Consume a nutrient-dense, anti-inflammatory diet. Fruits, vegetables, whole grains, and plant-based proteins should be prioritised.

To help reduce inflammation, include meals high in omega-3 fatty acids, such as flaxseeds, chia seeds, and fatty fish.

Exercise on a regular basis:

Exercise on a regular basis at a moderate intensity. Walking, swimming, and yoga are all activities that can help manage pain and enhance mood.

Consult a healthcare practitioner or a competent fitness expert to develop an activity regimen that is suited to your specific needs.

Adequate sleep and rest:

Make getting adequate sleep each night a priority. Quality sleep is critical for stress management and general wellness.

Create a relaxing sleep environment by establishing a nighttime routine.

Stress Reduction:

Meditation, deep breathing exercises, and mindfulness are all stress-reduction approaches.

Consider combining stress-relieving hobbies you like, such as reading, listening to music, or spending time in nature.

Hydration:

Drink lots of water throughout the day to stay hydrated.

Caffeine and alcohol should be avoided since they may aggravate symptoms.

Regular Medical Exams:

Maintain frequent check-ups with your healthcare practitioner and explain any changes in symptoms.

Manage your treatment plan in collaboration with your healthcare team.

Techniques for Pain Management:

Consider non-pharmacological pain relief methods such as heat treatment, acupuncture, or physical therapy.

Find appropriate pain relief options in collaboration with your healthcare physician.

The Mind-Body Connection

To encourage relaxation and strengthen the mind-body connection, consider mind-body techniques such as meditation, yoga, or tai chi.

Participate in support groups or therapy to connect with individuals who understand your situation.

Holistic Treatments:

Under the supervision of experienced practitioners, try alternative therapies such as acupuncture, chiropractic care, or massage therapy.

Prepare Yourself:

Keep up to date with endometriosis and its treatment options. Knowledge enables you to make educated health decisions.

By speaking freely with your healthcare staff, you can advocate for yourself.

Work-Life Integration:

Achieve a good work-life balance. Manage your workload and, if necessary, seek accommodations.

Inform your employer about your illness in order to create a supportive work atmosphere.

Remember that everyone with endometriosis has a different experience, and what works for one person may not work for another.

10 Day Meal Planning for Endometriosis

Day 1:

Breakfast: Smoothie with kale, banana, frozen berries, chia seeds, and almond milk.

Lunch: Quinoa salad with roasted vegetables, chickpeas, and a lemon-tahini dressing.

Dinner: Lentil and vegetable stew with sweet potato.

Snack: Guacamole and Vegetable Sticks

Day 2:

Breakfast: Overnight chia seed pudding with almond milk, topped with sliced strawberries and shredded coconut.

Lunch: Chickpea and vegetable curry with brown rice.

Dinner: Zucchini noodles with tomato sauce and roasted chickpeas.

Snack: Turmeric Roasted Cauliflower

Day 3:

Breakfast: Oatmeal topped with sliced banana, walnuts, and a drizzle of maple syrup.

Lunch: Spinach and arugula salad with roasted beets, quinoa, and balsamic vinaigrette.

Dinner: Stuffed bell peppers with quinoa, black beans, corn, and salsa.

Snack: Greek yogurt with a sprinkle of granola.

Day 4:

Breakfast: Vegan avocado toast with cherry tomatoes and a sprinkle of nutritional yeast.

Lunch: Hummus and veggie wrap with whole grain tortilla, cucumber, bell peppers, and mixed greens.

Dinner: Eggplant and chickpea curry with basmati rice.

Snack: Trail mix (nuts, seeds, and dried fruits).

Day 5:

Breakfast: Acai bowl with granola, mixed berries, and a drizzle of almond butter.

Lunch: Roasted vegetable and quinoa bowl with tahini dressing.

Dinner: Vegan lentil and mushroom lasagna.

Snack: Edamame with sea salt.

Day 6:

Breakfast: Green smoothie with spinach, pineapple, banana, and coconut water.

Lunch: Avocado and black bean burrito bowl with cilantro lime rice.

Dinner: Vegan sweet potato and black bean enchiladas.

Snack: Rice cakes with avocado slices

Day 7:

Breakfast: Vegan blueberry pancakes with maple syrup.

Lunch: Mediterranean chickpea salad with tomatoes, cucumbers, olives, and a lemon-tahini dressing.

Dinner: Vegan cauliflower and chickpea curry with brown rice.

Snack: Fresh fruit salad.

Day 8:

Breakfast: Vegan protein smoothie with pea protein powder, almond milk, mixed berries, and a tablespoon of almond butter.

Lunch: Quinoa and kale stuffed acorn squash with cranberries and pecans.

Dinner: Vegan stir-fry with tofu, broccoli, bell peppers, and a soy-ginger sauce.

Snack: Frozen grapes.

Day 9:

Breakfast: Vegan banana walnut muffins with a side of fruit.

Lunch: Vegan black bean and corn salad with lime vinaigrette.

Dinner: Vegan chickpea and vegetable stir-fry with quinoa.

Snack: Hummus with carrot sticks.

Day 10:

Breakfast: Vegan protein smoothie bowl with spinach, frozen berries, chia seeds, and almond milk.

Lunch: Vegan Buddha bowl with quinoa, roasted sweet potato, kale, avocado, and tahini dressing.

Dinner: Vegan lentil and vegetable curry with basmati rice.

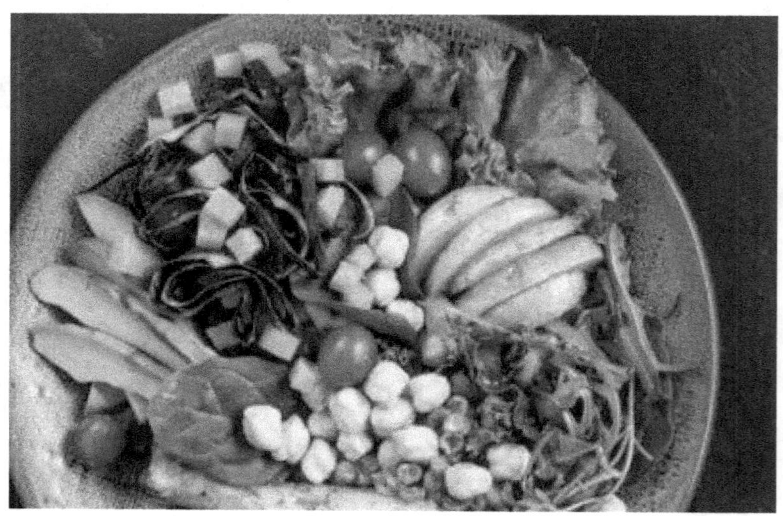

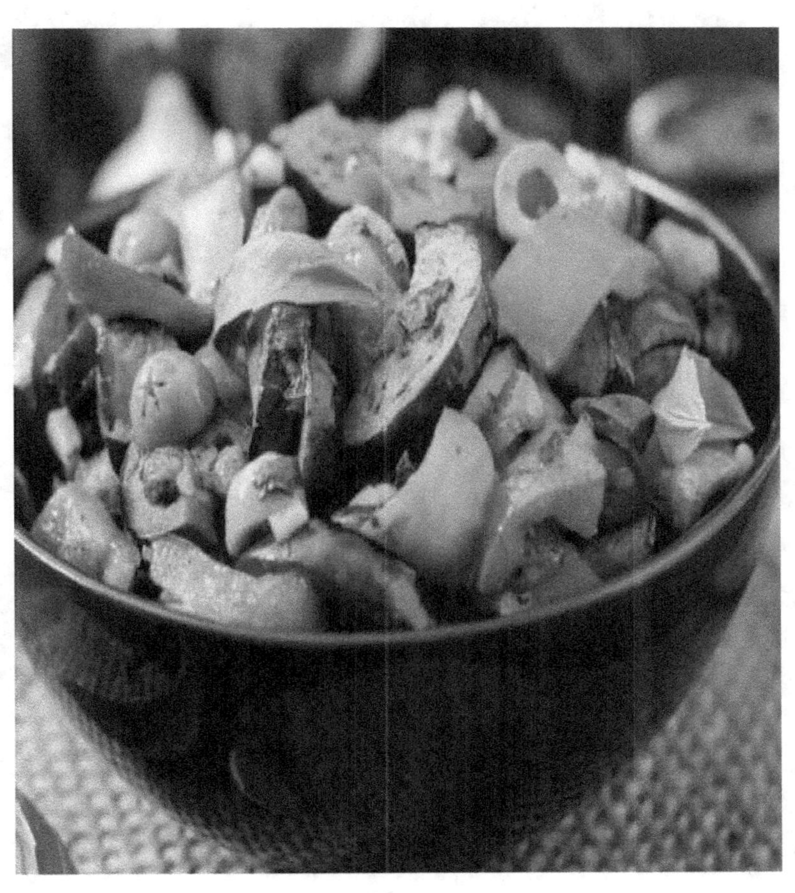

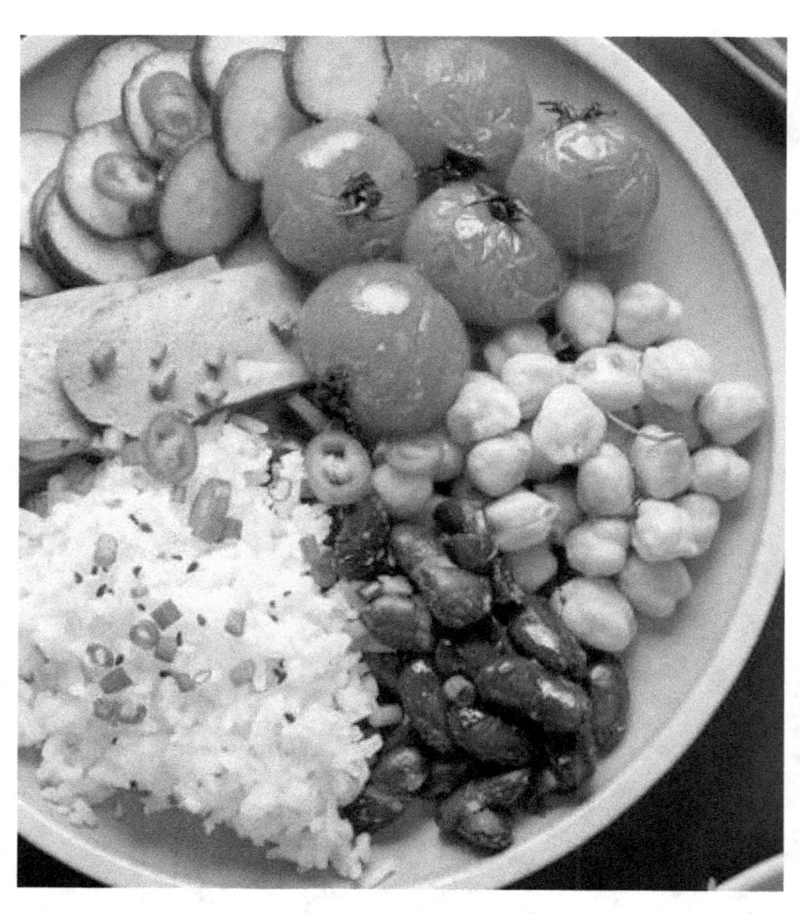

CHAPTER 9: CONCLUSION

The Endometriosis Plant-Based Diet Cookbook is a thorough handbook and a source of empowerment for anyone dealing with endometriosis. This culinary adventure, rich in delectable and healthy plant-based foods, is more than just a collection of recipes; it is a testament to the transformational power of taking a holistic approach to managing this difficult disease.

The meticulously crafted dishes not only prioritise the principles of a plant-based diet, but also deliberately contain anti-inflammatory elements. By emphasising the advantages of whole foods, the cookbook corresponds with a growing body of evidence indicating that dietary choices can play an important part in alleviating endometriosis symptoms.

Beyond the kitchen, the cookbook promotes a lifestyle change by emphasising the interdependence of nutrition, mental health, and general wellness. Each dish is a gastronomic festival, providing folks with a variety of flavours that not only satisfy the taste senses but also contribute to the overarching objective of maintaining hormonal balance and lowering inflammation.

Furthermore, the addition of instructive sections about endometriosis, nutrition, and practical cooking advice increases the cookbook's usefulness as a holistic resource. It not only provides folks with tasty and healthy food, but it also transmits information, encouraging a sense of agency in health management.

In essence, the Endometriosis Plant-Based Diet Cookbook emerges not just as a culinary guide, but also as a caring companion on the path to wellness.

STAY HEALTHY!

Bonus

MEAL PLANNER
DAILY
DATE
BREAKFAST
NOTES
LUNCH
SNACK
ITEMS LIST
DINNER

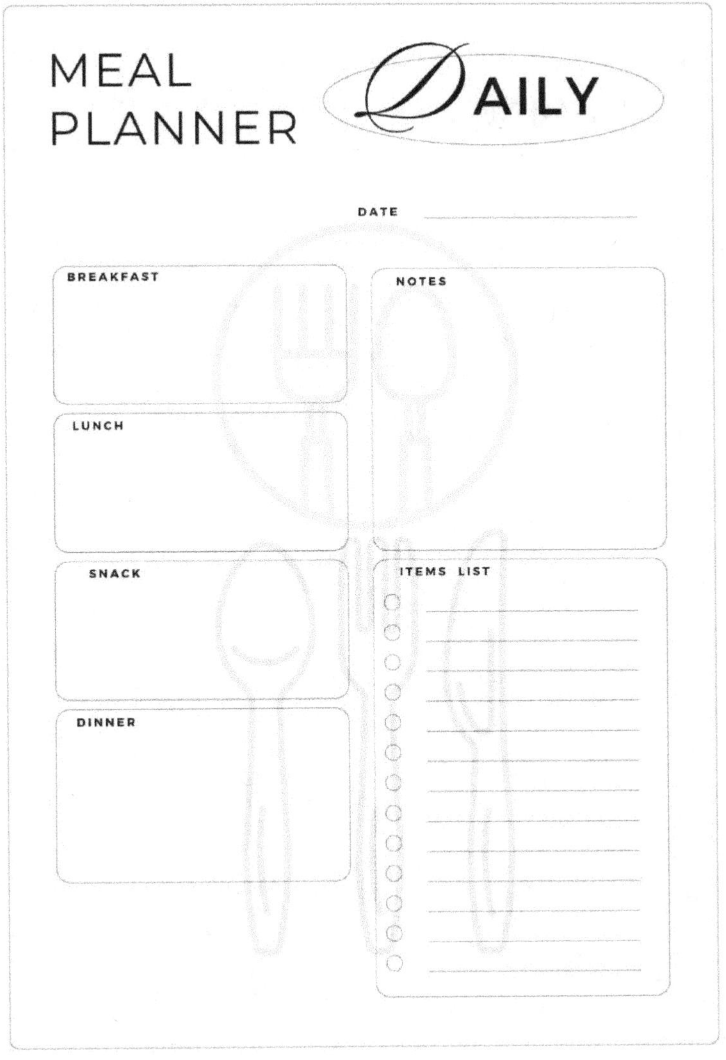

MEAL PLANNER

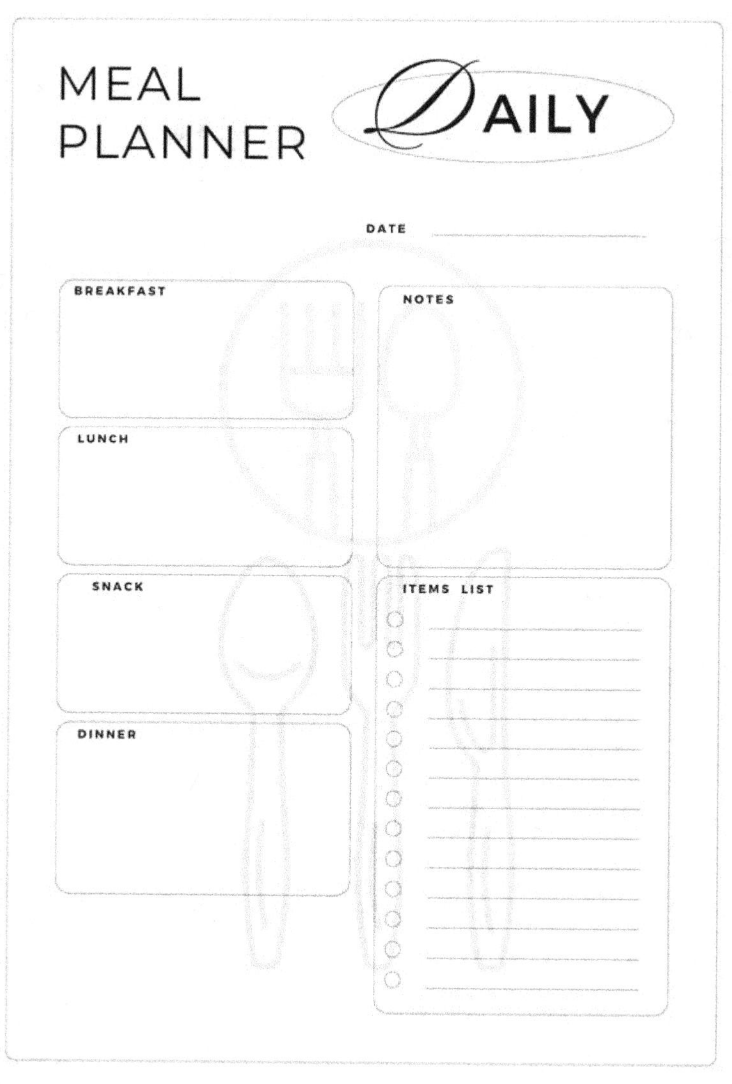

MEAL PLANNER

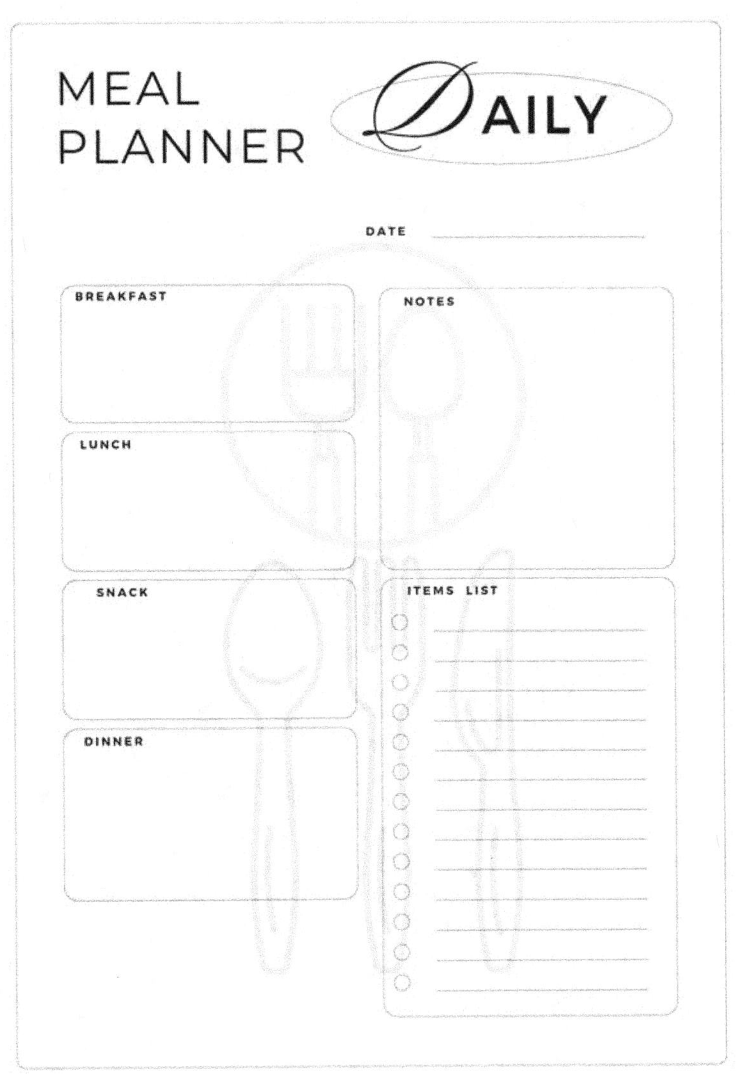

DAILY

DATE

BREAKFAST

NOTES

LUNCH

SNACK

ITEMS LIST

DINNER

MEAL PLANNER

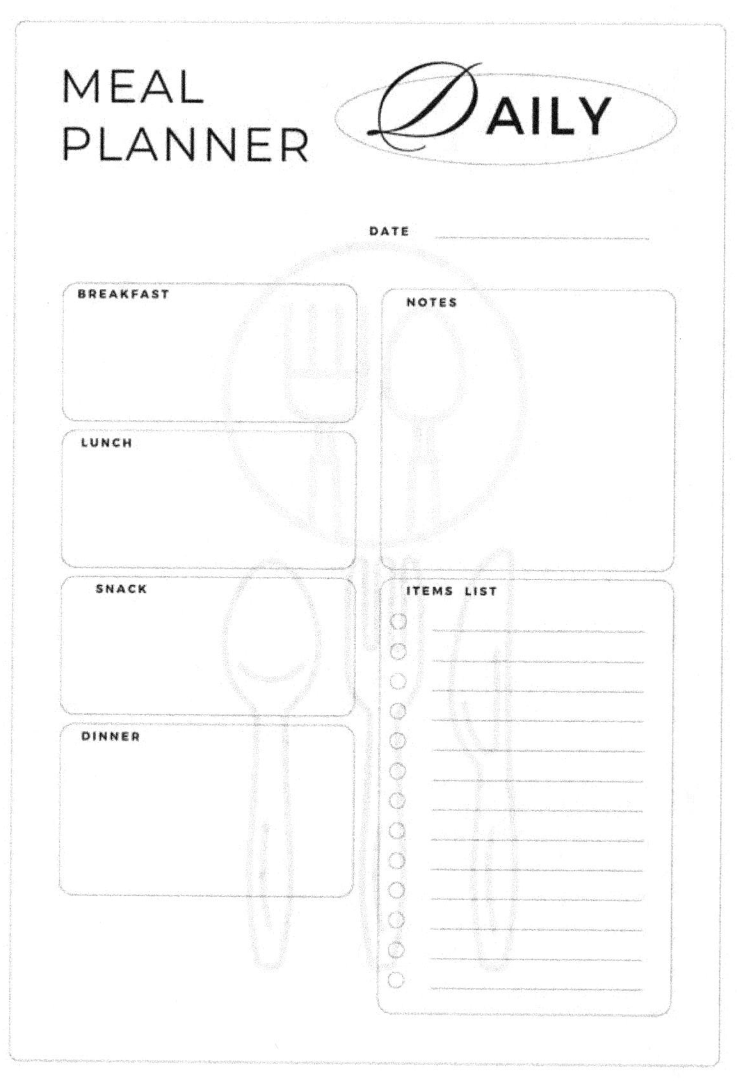

DAILY

DATE

BREAKFAST

NOTES

LUNCH

SNACK

ITEMS LIST

DINNER

MEAL PLANNER

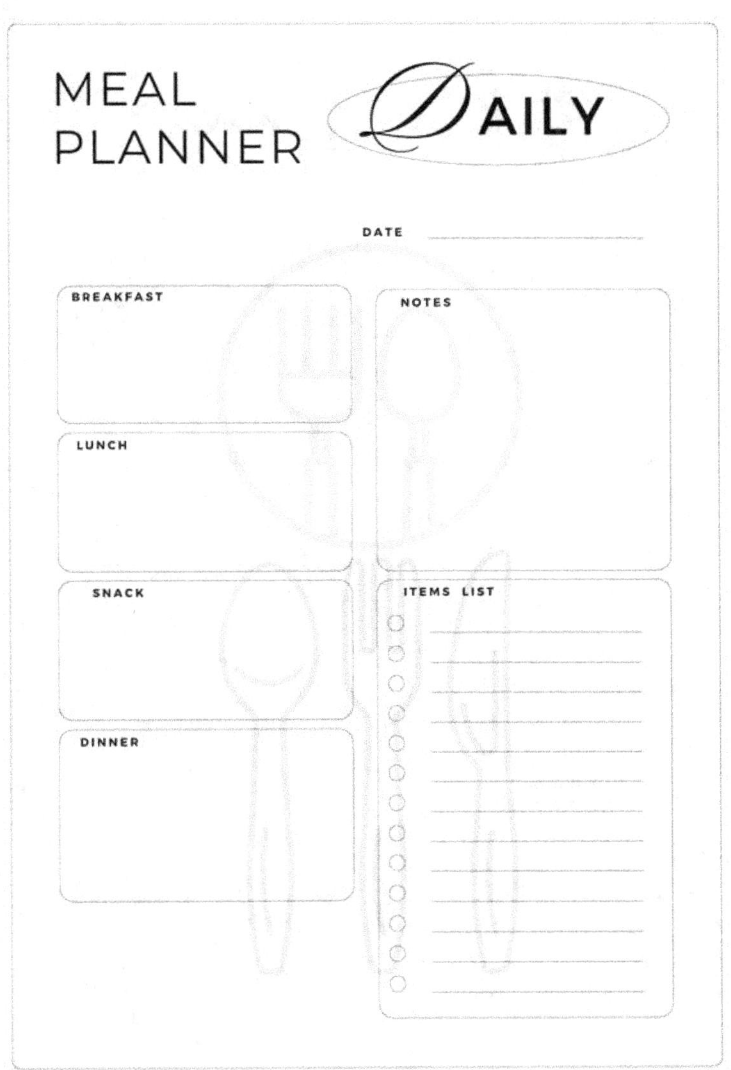

DAILY

DATE _______________

BREAKFAST

LUNCH

SNACK

DINNER

NOTES

ITEMS LIST

MEAL PLANNER

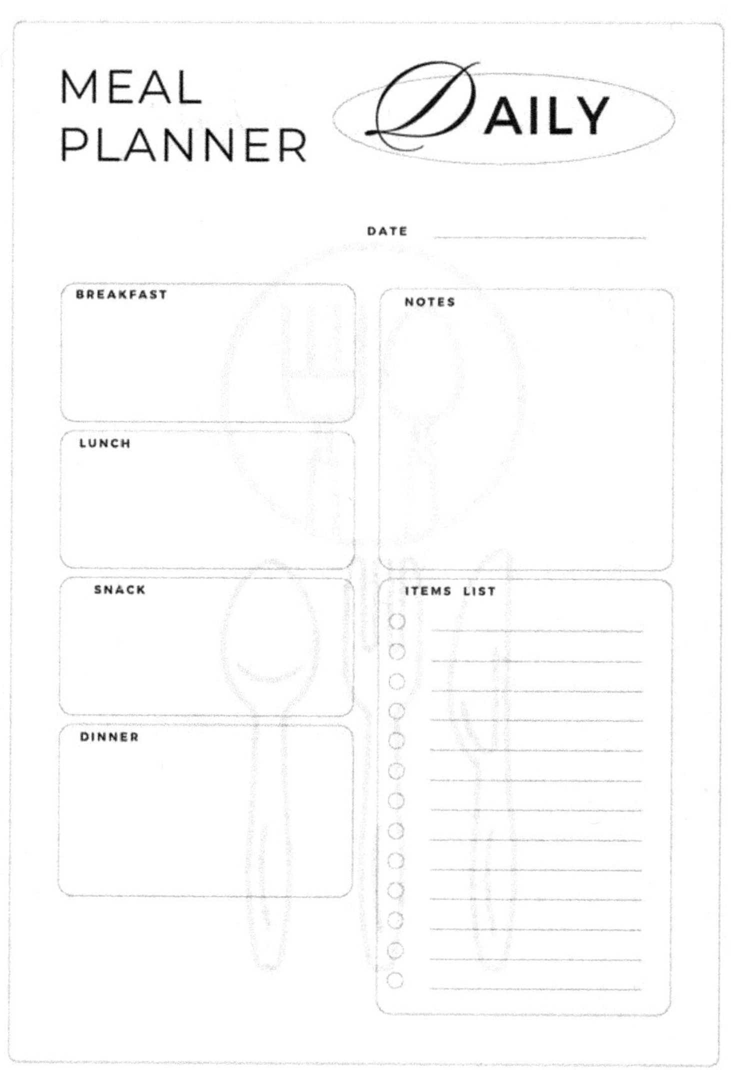

DAILY

DATE

BREAKFAST

LUNCH

SNACK

DINNER

NOTES

ITEMS LIST

MEAL PLANNER

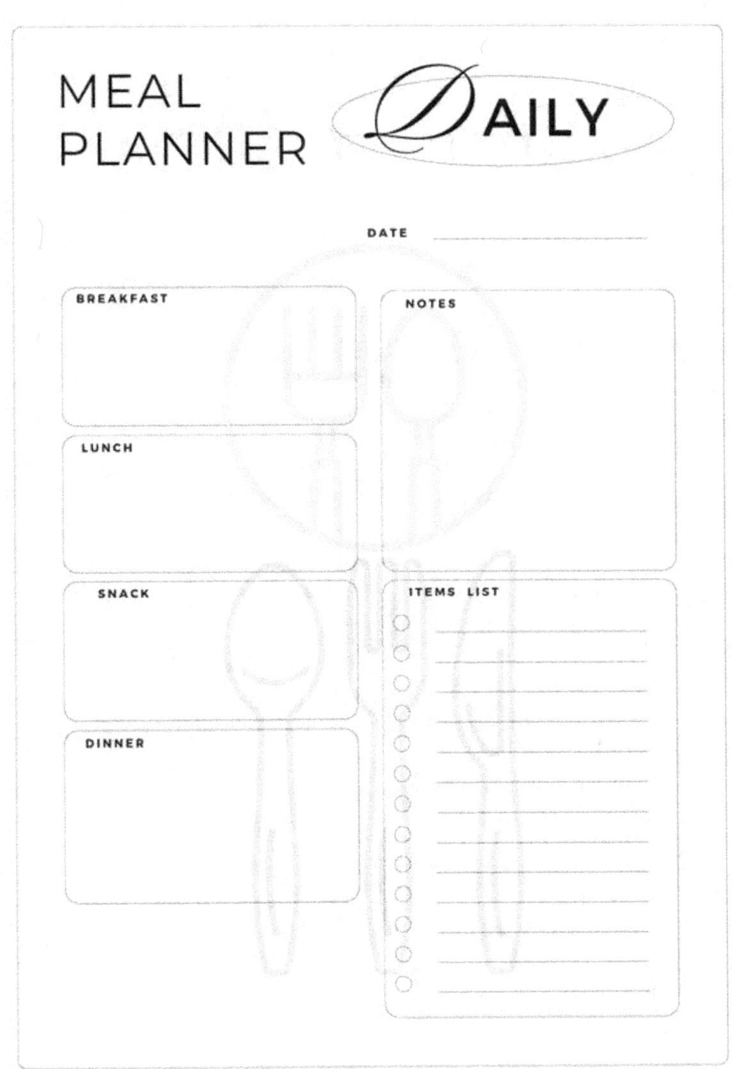

DAILY

DATE ___________

BREAKFAST

LUNCH

SNACK

DINNER

NOTES

ITEMS LIST

MEAL PLANNER

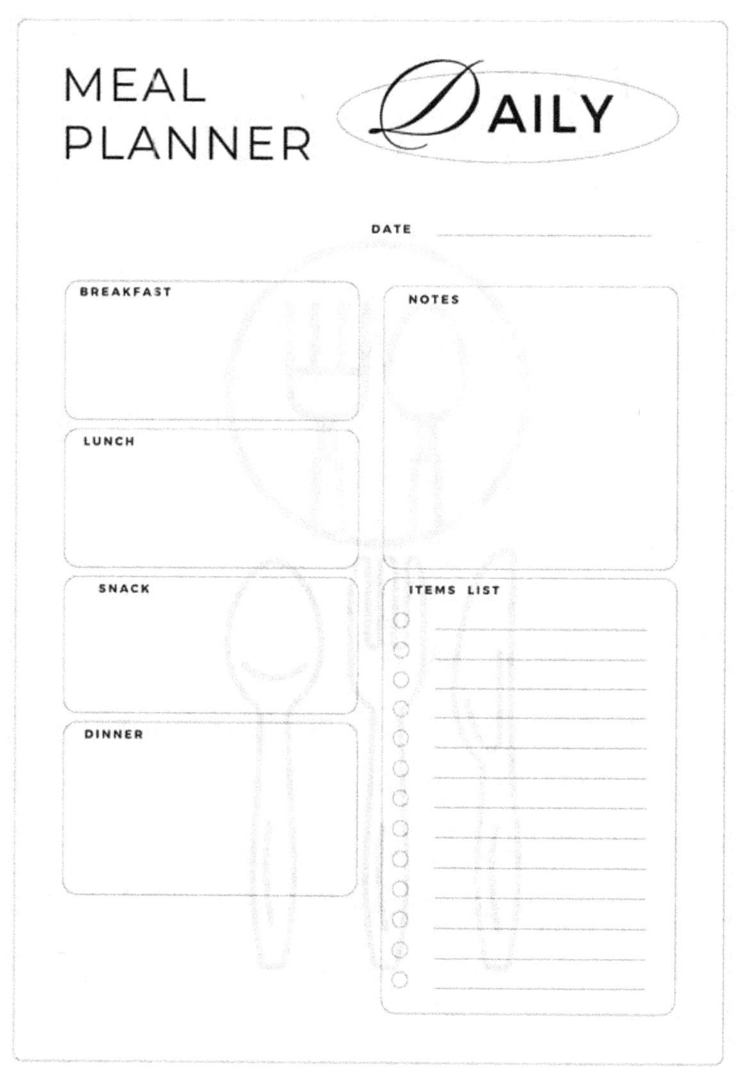

DAILY

DATE ___________

BREAKFAST

LUNCH

SNACK

DINNER

NOTES

ITEMS LIST

MEAL PLANNER

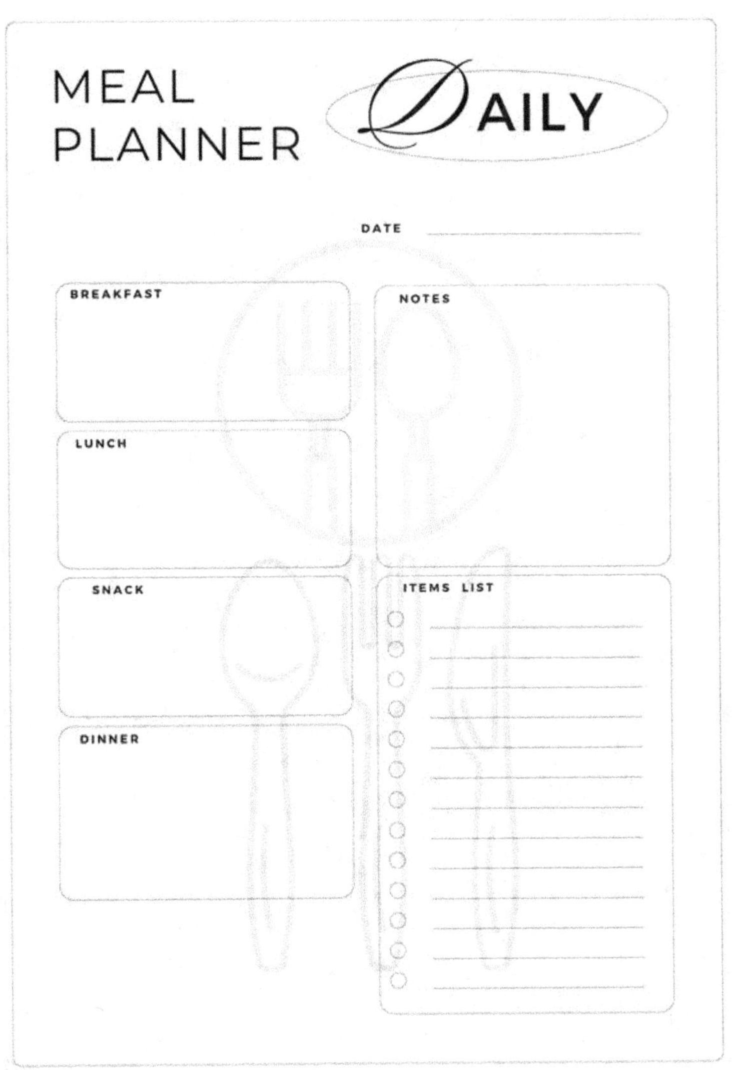

MEAL PLANNER

$\mathcal{D}$AILY

DATE _______________

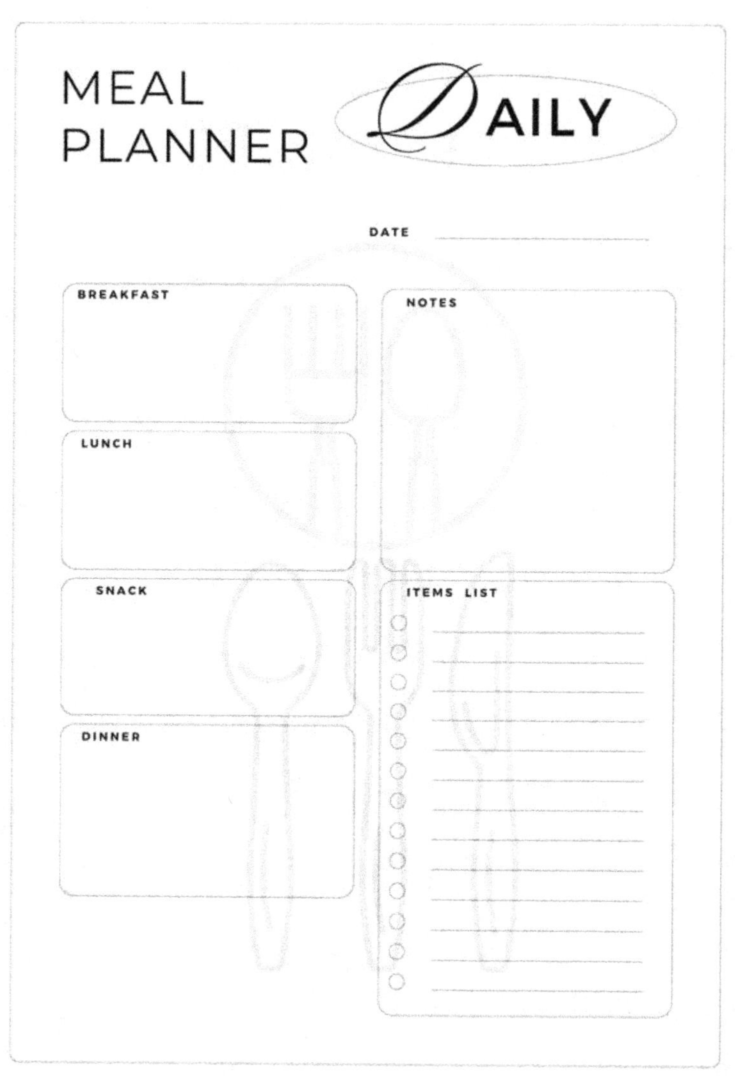

BREAKFAST

LUNCH

SNACK

DINNER

NOTES

ITEMS LIST